A CATHOLIC VIEW OF HOLISM

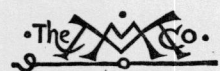

THE MACMILLAN COMPANY
NEW YORK · BOSTON · CHICAGO · DALLAS
ATLANTA · SAN FRANCISCO

MACMILLAN & CO., LIMITED
LONDON · BOMBAY · CALCUTTA
MELBOURNE

THE MACMILLAN CO. OF CANADA, LTD.
TORONTO

A CATHOLIC VIEW OF HOLISM

A criticism of the theory put forward by General Smuts in his book, "Holism and Evolution"

BY

MONSIGNOR KOLBE, D.D., D.LITT.
OF THE UNIVERSITY OF CAPE TOWN

WITH A FOREWORD BY THE
RIGHT HONOURABLE GENERAL SMUTS

NEW YORK
THE MACMILLAN COMPANY
1928

All rights reserved

Copyright, 1928,
By THE MACMILLAN COMPANY

Set up and printed
Published, March, 1928

PRINTED IN THE UNITED STATES

Nihil Obstat
 ARTHUR J. SCANLAN, S.T.D.
  Censor Librorum.

Imprimatur
 ✠ PATRICK CARDINAL HAYES
  Archbishop, New York.

New York, April 7, 1928.

FOREWORD

THIS criticism of my work *Holism and Evolution* will be of interest not only to readers of that book, but also to many others who feel attracted by the central idea of Holism. Mgr. Kolbe's valuable Essay is more than a criticism of my book, although from that point of view too it is very well worth reading. It is in some respects a supplement to my book; it fills certain gaps in it; and it shows the importance of the main idea for religion. Mgr. Kolbe shows that the idea (in its Aristotelian garb) played a great part in the philosophy of the Middle Ages until, in the seventeenth century, the rise of the Cartesian system gave a new direction to philosophy. He suggests the view that Holism is a return to the older, saner outlook which has during the last three centuries been pushed into the background by the mechanistic worldview of Descartes. All this he does with full and profound knowledge, in clear and picturesque language, and with a constructive aim which makes his Essay specially valuable. Although it professes to set forth the Catholic view-point, and contains some pointed warnings against my heresies, its appeal is, in fact, more general, and it will interest a much wider circle than the Catholic community.

It was a matter of great gratification to me that, on the appearance of *Holism,* Mgr. Kolbe at once acknowledged himself a Holist. I hailed him as a convert. There I was wrong, and he has written this interesting Essay to prove that Holism is older than my book, that it is at least as old as Christianity, and that St. Paul was the greatest Holist of them all. So be it. I waive all claim to priority before such august competition.

What is of most significance in this connection is that to Mgr. Kolbe, as to me, Holism is more than a mere abstract idea, a new item of speculation to tickle the interest of the schools. To him as to me it is instinct with reality, a great central truth which illuminates all other truths. He sees clearly the scientific and philosophic importance of the concept, he realises what a transforming power it is bound to exercise over the most general view-points in science and philosophy. But above all he is conscious of its profound significance in the domain of religion. The word Holism stirs strange depths in him, it raises for him the image of that redeemed, transfigured universe of St. Paul's great language, in which "God will be all in all"—or Holism finally consummated.

This, of course, is an aspect of Holism which is not touched upon in my book. I was there trying to lay the foundations of the idea; I was trying to build the new structure from its foundations. The Religious Ideal, like the other great Ideals and Values of the spirit, is not yet reached in my treatment of Holism, although, to be sure, the understanding reader will find more in the book than is actually written there. Now from this religious point of view, and especially to guard against any misunderstanding of the Catholic position, Mgr. Kolbe feels called upon to state explicitly what is not directly set out in my book. Within the limited scientific purview of the book I do not discuss God, as such a discussion would in my opinion have been out of place in such a context. But Mgr. Kolbe holds that from the Catholic point of view not even a scientific statement of the universe is correct which does not make explicit reference to the First Cause which underlies and sustains all secondary or particular causes. No account of the finite universe is for him true which omits its relation to the infinite. And he wishes to guard against the view which might possibly consider such relation or reference as unfounded, and the infinite as therefore unnecessary surplusage in a scientific scheme. Not that he attributes such a view to me, but he wishes to prevent others from wrongly inferring such a view from my silence.

My silence on this point is, as I have said, due to the limited introductory scope of my book. In my development of Holism I have not yet come to the consideration of such subjects as the infinite. And yet even so, the relation of the finite to the infinite is implicit in all that I say in regard to the whole. My treatment of Holism is destructive of the self-sufficiency of the particular or the finite. The popular view of the finite particular or "thing" I show to be a false abstraction, and I correct the false simplification involved by the introduction of the concept of the field. Nothing is complete in itself or sufficient unto itself. The finite endures in the communion of the infinite. Holism by its very nature denies reality to the particular by itself and in itself and apart from the context of its field. The religious aspect of this truth to which Mgr. Kolbe draws attention seems to me to be implied in the concept of Holism as I have expounded it. And indeed nowhere is the power of this concept demonstrated more clearly and forcibly than in the way in which the most far-reaching and important distinctions of philosophical and religious thought are seen to flow quite simply and naturally from it as a centre. But in my book all this is still more or less implicit, and the task of explicit development has still to be undertaken.

It is not the least valuable service of Mgr. Kolbe's Essay that it shows that there are these wider and important implications and applications of the Holistic conception still to be drawn and made. His discriminating support, from his own angle and with his great weight, is very welcome and encouraging to me. That a fellow South African, so outstanding in every way, has so soon responded to the appeal of Holism is to me a sign that in writing my book in this far-off corner of the world I have not been a voice crying in the wilderness.

J. C. SMUTS.

AUTHOR'S PREFACE

THIS Essay originally appeared as a series of articles in the weekly press of Cape Town —one in *The Cape* and the rest in *The Southern Cross*. They are left substantially unaltered, though doubtless a little polishing would be an improvement. There is a freshness about journalistic work which perhaps compensates for the absence of tricks of scholarship.

There are, however, those who demand at least references where great names are appealed to. For such information I refer readers to Canon Dorlodot's *Darwinism and Catholic Thought* (Burns, Oates and Washbourne, Ltd.), where the teaching of St. Basil and St. Augustine is fully investigated.

I do not claim any representative position,

but speak for myself only, and indicate the fact by using "a" instead of "the" in my title.

It is impossible to find words to express my appreciation of the generous and good-humoured Foreword which General Smuts allows me to print. It made me want to cancel a great deal of my criticism; but I have left it all in because it enhances the generosity of the Foreword. Apart from all criticism, readers of *Holism and Evolution* will be glad to have this brief but important pronouncement on the philosophical view-point of its distinguished author.

F. C. KOLBE.

Cape Town,
March 25, 1927.

CONTENTS

CHAP.		PAGE
	PRELIMINARY	1
I.	THE THEORY	7
II.	MAPPING OUT THE CAMPAIGN	12
III.	BACKWARD STEPS	17
IV.	THE POSITION BEFORE AND AFTER DARWIN	23
V.	CAN THE INFINITE BE IGNORED?	28
VI.	STAGES OF EVOLUTION	33
VII.	BRIDGING THE GAPS	39
VIII.	SENSE AND REASON	45
IX.	THE THREEFOLD CREATIVE WORD	51
X.	WHAT IS HOLISM?	56
XI.	IS THE CELL THE UNIT OF ORGANIC LIFE?	62
XII.	"WHOLES" AND "SUBSTANTIAL FORMS"	72
XIII.	THE THEORY OF RELATIVITY	77
XIV.	THE MORAL ASPECT OF HOLISM	84
XV.	EXTREME CASES	91
XVI.	THE SUPREME WHOLE OR FORM	98

A CATHOLIC VIEW OF HOLISM

PRELIMINARY

"HOLISM AND EVOLUTION"
(PEEPS INTO THE WORLD OF ART)

SOME folk might think, on comparing my title with its parallel heading, that I have fallen into an inconsistency. What has scientific philosophy to do with art? My answer to this consists in the contention, which I never weary of stressing, that recent times have unduly narrowed the conception of art as compared with that of the Greeks and of the medieval thinkers. Any and every output of human energy which consciously aims at excellence is of the nature of art. It may be intellectual: it may be moral: it may be imaginative: it may be creative for the eye or for the ear. If there is design for the expression of an idea, it is art. A speech of Demosthenes is a work of art for its mental and emotional persuasiveness, and its elegance and even profusion of language is appropriate to its aim. Kant's *Critique* is a work of art, although his literary style is heavy. It is possible, therefore, for a treatise on scientific philosophy to have a rightful place in the art world either because of the ingenuity and skill of its persuasive or architectonic structure or because of its appropriate literary elegance. General Smuts's *Holism and Evolution* has both these qualities.

With the truth of the theory in this remarkable book I am not here immediately concerned. I discuss it later on. But the presentment of the theory is a model of intellectual persuasiveness. A basic idea for the explanation of the phenomena of the visible world has been found and clearly stated. It is steadily applied through all the stages from the primeval fire-mist to the highest products of life. The idea is that evolution is *creative,* that is to say, each forward move in the process results in a new *totum* or whole (hence, from the Greek, the name Holism), which is something more than the sum total of the constituent parts. The way in which the entire argument is mapped out, points of vantage seized, troops of illustrations deployed, reserves marched up at critical moments, reminds one of a military campaign. General Smuts has a strategic mind.

All this is laid before us with unusual clarity of style. Only one sentence in the book did I have to read over again to catch its sense. There is, perhaps, more repetition than elegance demands; but one has to hit a nail often to drive it into hard wood, and here at least the nail is always hit right on the head. This leads us to pass from argumentative to literary qualities. For sheer English this book is an outstanding addition to South African literature. I was glad to see that Senator Langenhoven has recognised this and has expressed his pride in the achievement. Little flaws might be pointed out, as might be expected from the extraordinary speed with which the work must have been written. Purists will smile at the Afrikanderism "just now"—the familiar *net nou*. Pedants might object to an occasional disregard of the English idiomatic use of *shall* and *will*—that delicacy in the expression of futurity which belongs to English alone, but which is now commonly violated even in England itself. But these are trifles. The English in this book is always appropriate to the subject, is not over-loaded with irrelevant ornament, but rises from time to time as wider vistas open up before the writer. There is a simple, solid and dignified passage of eloquence at the very end, worthy of a place of honour in any literature. It is too long to quote here in its entirety, but it begins thus:—

"The reflections embodied in this work lie far removed from the busy and exciting scenes in which most of my life has been spent, and yet both of them tend towards the same general conclusions. It has been my lot to have passed many of the years of my life amid the conflicts of men, in their wars and their council chambers. Everywhere I have seen men search and struggle for the good with grim determination and earnestness, and with a sincerity of purpose which added to the poignancy of the fratricidal strife. But we are still far, very far, from the goal to which holism points. The Great War—with its infinite loss and suffering, its toll of untold lives, the shattering of great States and almost of civilisation, the fearful waste of goodwill and sincere human ideals which followed the close of that vast tragedy—has been proof enough for our day and generation that we are yet far off the attainment of the ideal of a really holistic universe. But everywhere, too, I have seen that it was at bottom a struggle for the good, a wild striving towards human betterment: that blindly, and through blinding mists of passions and illusions, men are yet sincerely, earnestly groping towards the light, towards the ideal of a better, more secure life for themselves and for their fellows."

Whether we agree with the theory or not, we can hail the book as something that permanently lifts the level of South African literature. It may be difficult reading, but it is worth a thousand novels.

CHAPTER I

THE THEORY

MANY years ago, when I was examining in Philosophy, a very thoughtful set of papers was sent in by a student of Stellenbosch. If we could only foresee, "if we could look into the seeds of time and say which grain will grow and which will not," I should have read those papers with far greater interest than I did. For the name of the student was Jan Smuts. Other students in various years sent in papers equally good, one at least much better, but their philosophical education seems to have ended there. They have not fulfilled their promise. They reproduced the thoughts of others, sometimes with great skill; but they did not *think*. Jan Smuts started with a handicap. His professor was a dear old man without a germ of originality and hardly a gleam of humour, who handled a text-book of undisguised materialism, covering it with a camouflage of genuine but emotional piety, "spreading a compost o'er the weeds," as Shakespeare says. But the germs of thought were there, and now this Stellenbosch student, despite a strenuous career of active strife in field and forum, has sent forth a volume which will extend the thinking powers of students in every University in the world. It is a phenomenon of intense interest to us in South Africa.

A true thinker will think even on a battle-field and amid the arid wastes of political oratory, but this book is the fruit of wide reading and intense scientific study, and required years of laborious writing. Where did he get the time? When a couple of years ago General Smuts was elected President of the Science Association, many thought it was merely a political honour and expected nothing from his inaugural address but scientific platitudes. They were surprised. They have much more reason to be surprised now. For this is an original, intensive and comprehensive explanation of the whole course of the visible world from the primeval fire-mist to the highest human civilisation. It is a view which challenges, and must receive, the most careful consideration.

A superficial judgment might put General Smuts down as a materialist. He seems to say that matter has *in itself* a creative power which enables it to rise through stage after stage of being until it reaches the spiritual. But he does not discuss the phrase "in itself," and he explains creativeness merely as a bringing about a state of things that was not there before. If you ask him how matter got its creative power, or what place the idea of the Creator has in His scheme, he says he is writing Scientific Philosophy, not Metaphysics or Natural Theology. Yet he will be accused. "Fundamentalism" will anathematise him. He would not be allowed to teach in Dayton. It is not so, however. Much as we shall have to differ from him here or there, we admit from the first his high spiritual aim. He might almost have taken as a subtitle for his book, "A way of escape from mechanistic and materialistic views."

When declining to consider the conception of creation in the strict sense, *i.e.* out of nothing, General Smuts uses an unfortunate word —a rare thing with him—and says it is "unintelligible." Being an infinite act it is, of course, incomprehensible, but that is a different word altogether. The former word, in its usage at least, connotes "*against* reason;" the latter implies "*above* reason." Probably all that was meant was "not within the bounds of our experience."

In order to make my criticism more intelligible, I shall take a leaf out of the book of our theologians who often prefix a "Status quæstionis" to a thesis. I will map out the field before starting the campaign. This will occupy me next time. Meanwhile I say now that most of the confusion of thought that has obsessed recent philosophies has come from the revolt of Descartes, who made a complete severance between soul and body. This resulted in sheer materialism in Science and in strange acrobatic feats in Philosophy. There are many converging signs that a counter-revolution is in progress. The *Times Literary Supplement* lately headed its chief article with the title, "The Dethronement of Descartes." The significance of General Smuts's book is that it comes at a crisis in the battle and will probably complete the rout. Like Milton's chanticleer it utters a clarion note which scatters the rear of darkness thin. As a philosophy Cartesianism is dead, and people are beginning to ask, "Was there then some life in what it revolted from?"

CHAPTER II

MAPPING OUT THE CAMPAIGN

WESTERN civilisation, which is gradually becoming universal, is the result of three tendencies—Oriental (contemplative), Greek (speculative) and Roman (organising)—Oriental mysticism, Greek philosophy and Roman law and order. These tendencies at first lay side by side with very little commingling. But when the Christian Idea came into the world, it seized upon all three and incorporated them into itself. And this union was, to use a scientific metaphor, not a mechanical mixture but a chemical combination. As General Smuts would put it, it was *creative,* forming a new *totum* or whole, transcending while utilising all the three constituent parts, animating them like a soul and not merely joining them as in partnership. The best individual type of the union is St. Paul, who was Hebrew and Greek and Roman, but all Christian. We shall return to this point when answering General Smuts's passing criticism on Catholic asceticism, which he takes to be merely Oriental.

Scientific Philosophy, then, began with the Greeks, and from the first they fastened on to the idea of Evolution. Many and wild were the guesses they made, some of them extraordinarily acute and penetrating. It was the first, and premature, stage of the Evolution Theory. Owing to their inevitable lack of accumulated scientific fact, they accomplished nothing but the creation of the art of dialectics, and this art produced the men called Sophists. Failure seemed imminent. Then it was that Socrates intervened and turned the thoughts of men from baseless speculations to fruitful self-study and discipline. Evolution went into the background, and had to wait till the world was readier.

When the Christian Idea came, its first efforts towards self-expression were naturally and necessarily concerned with Faith. But the Idea is a universal one and compels thought in every direction. What would it say about Evolution? It must be borne in mind that there was a continuity between the Pagan and the Christian intellectual activities. There were still Universities, and Christians studied in them. The question was bound to arise about the origin of the world, and its relations to the Infinite. There was Scripture to interpret. It is a surprise to many moderns that the deepest minds among the Church Fathers, like St. Basil for the East and St. Augustine for the West, adopted the idea of Absolute Evolution. There was first the conception of the Infinite, to which Plato and Aristotle had already attained. In God there is no succession or time. A moment or a billion years, it is all the same to Him. The early Christian philosophers therefore considered that the revealed mode of creation was a poetic and

Oriental way of accommodating incomprehensible truth to finite minds. God's act, simple in itself, is successive and graduated to us. They held, therefore, that the Creator by a single word, which was to reverberate and actuate throughout the ages, brought into existence a mass of unformed matter and endowed it with the power of forming itself into higher and higher substances, until it should reach even the body of man. The forms of inorganic substances and the souls of vegetable and animal beings were "educed from the potentiality of matter itself." Matter was endowed with *seminales rationes* (creative qualities), said St. Basil and St. Augustine. The Creator did not need to keep on intervening to supply for insufficiencies in His work. When it comes to the *soul* of man and to questions of Grace, a wholly different question arises.

I say that many are surprised at being told this. But they need not be quite so much surprised if they will only remember the sympathetic creativeness that St. Paul attributes to the material world. "For the expectation of the creature (creation) waiteth for the revelation of the sons of God. For the creature was made subject to vanity, not willingly, but by reason of him that made it subject, in hope. Because the creature also itself shall be delivered from the servitude of corruption, into the liberty of the glory of the children of God. For we know that every creature (all creation) groaneth and travaileth (with maternal creativeness) in pain, even till now."

How "Special Creation" and "Fixity of Species" ever came to be regarded as the orthodox position will be considered next time. Already it is evident that a wide range of agreement is possible for us with Evolution as presented by General Smuts. The reason why Catholic philosophers have not all gone as far as St. Basil and St. Augustine is chiefly the scientific fact that, in spite of the most eager investigation, spontaneous generation has not been proved. Scientists can hardly blame us for not outrunning our facts.

CHAPTER III

BACKWARD STEPS

We have seen that the first stage of Evolution Theories consisted in the premature but not altogether futile speculations of the Greeks. The second stage was the Christian synthesis of four ideas: (1) the conception of the visible world as a stream of phenomena (*panta rhei,* as the old sage put it, "it is all a flow"); (2) the Greek intellectual presentment of the Infinite; (3) the Hebrew concept of the world as the *voice* of God; (4) the revelation in Genesis of creation *ex nihilo.* In the Infinite there is no time, no succession, "no shadow of alteration." The one Word which produced, produces and sustains the universe is indefinitely varied from our point of view, but it is an unbroken unity in God. Rightly, therefore, when we are not by way of being philosophical, do we accept the poetry and the analogies whereby our revelation of God and His ways has been made known to us. There are things better than philosophy. Indeed, philosophy is dangerous to those who do not know how to handle its tools.

The early Christian Philosophy, then, without disdaining the multiform simplicities of Scripture and ordinary life, which are just as true in their way as intellectual abstractions, laid down first that the Creative Word of God is in itself one and undivided, but that we, being conditioned by time and space, have not faculties to consider it directly so. The simplest refraction of this pure Divine ray is into three—(1) the Word creative of matter, (2) the Word creative of spiritual beings, (3) the Word creative of the supernatural. The study took on a new phase when this Word was made flesh and dwelt among us.

Here and now we are concerned with only

the first of the three ideas, *i.e.* the Word creative of matter, up to and perhaps even including the body of man. Sturdily true to their philosophical principles, St. Basil and St. Augustine saw no "jump" in the visible world which would have called for Divine "intervention" in the way of special creation. Neither spontaneous generation nor the wide reach from the worm to the elephant troubled them. The Creator sent matter into existence with all its potentialities, endowing it with some of His own creativeness, so that passing higher and higher from form to form it gave forth the voice that had caused it, and perpetually increased the volume of the chorus of creation's praise to its Maker.

How then did this clear view fall into abeyance? First of all, Philosophy and Theology had the great task of harmonising into system all the implications of the Christian Idea—a far higher work than the study of physical science. This reached its climax in the Summa of St. Thomas. For their science they looked to the scientists. And what were *they* doing? They were mostly absorbed in schemes of magic, swindling people with promises of the philosopher's stone to turn all things into gold, or with love philtres and poisons, or with the Elixir of Life. And now scientists have the brazen effrontery to blame the theologians for what was the fault of their own colleagues. One does not blame the Archbishop of Canterbury for not being a biologist. But even if the scientists had done their duty (and some of the theologians, like Albertus Magnus and Roger Bacon, began to show them the way), sufficient progress was not possible till such means as telescopes, microscopes, spectroscopes, etc., were available.

Even this dearth of knowledge might have been remedied, only then came the great upheaval. The Renaissance turned men's thoughts back to antiquity. The Fathers and the Scholastics, they said, wrote barbarous Latin. Medieval art was "Gothic." There was no language but Ciceronian Latin and

Platonic Greek. Philosophy and Theology went out of fashion. Luther's theories severed body and soul in religious thought. He maintained that what the body did could not affect the soul.

Then came Descartes, who, with the best intentions, for he was a devout Catholic, thought he could re-express all Philosophy from his own speculations. Among other things, he taught that the soul governed the body from without like an engine-driver. He even found a seat for the soul in the pineal gland. After that the old philosophy, though still taught in the Catholic Colleges, came to be by the "modernist" world looked upon as extinct.

But Descartes is dethroned, and the new school of Catholic Philosophy is now absorbing all the experience of the last four centuries and is restating the old solutions of the world's problems in modern ways. The scientists still talk as if it were extinct, but as a matter of fact it is taught in more Colleges and is held by more thinkers than any other system. It will prevail.

And now General Smuts has re-discovered part of it without knowing he has done so. That is why we find his book so interesting; and that is why we are going to be at such pains to say where we agree with him, and where we must part company.

CHAPTER IV

THE POSITION BEFORE AND AFTER DARWIN

WE have seen that the first phase of the Evolution Theory, that of the Greeks, was based, without much knowledge of Physical Science, on a philosophical attempt to unify the phenomena of the visible universe. The second, that of the early Christian philosophers, resulted from the union of Philosophy with Revelation, and was expressed as the Threefold Creative Word, originating and energising Matter, Spirit and Grace. The initial progress of Physical Science tended to break up this unity. Thinkers began to be frightened at the enormous jump between the worm and the elephant. The idea of special creation crept in. It had already begun even in St.

Augustine's time, and about it he dryly remarked that he could not see why we should want to postulate miracles at that stage of the world's existence. The mental confusion was greatly increased by the great disruption of the continuity of Philosophy and Religion, which culminated in Descartes' complete separation of Soul and Body in Man, and the consequent turning of all Physical Science into materialistic channels. The early pupils of Descartes—for the French are nothing if not logical—looked upon animals other than man as mere machines; they used to dissect cats and dogs alive, and laughed at their cries of pain as "the breaking up of the machinery." Many could see no bridge between one species and another and declared that when God wanted a cat or an oyster or a flea, He created one, or rather two, out of nothing. One brilliant genius postulated twenty-nine of St. Augustine's "miracles," without which the animal world could not have been set going. These ideas were called "Fixity of Species" and

"Special Creation." They never formed a part of Catholic Philosophy, and therefore amid the gibes of scientific evolutionists our withers are unwrung.

The rapid advance of science in the eighteenth and nineteenth centuries brought the Evolution Theory to its third phase, mainly in the person of Darwin. His view was almost entirely biological, and he accounted for the beginning of life by the special creation of one or a few initial germs. He found the jump from the inorganic to the organic more inexplicable than the far greater jump from Sense to Intelligence. He did not, of course, invent Evolution. He had predecessors. Development was in the air. What has given him his unique position is that he first so collocated, arranged and marshalled the facts as to show the plan of the world, and propounded laws governing the process of its growth. His laws were not adequate, but they were right as far as they went, and they justify us in placing him alongside of Copernicus and Newton as one of the great illuminators of scientific thought. His followers have broadened, and corrected, and amplified his views, and are still engaged in so doing, but they have not superseded him. They have also given Evolution a much stronger tendency to mechanistic materialism than he did. Trying to avoid the shadow of "creation" which Darwin postulated, one of his followers (who ought to have been put in a glass case and exhibited) suggested that the first germs of life came to earth in a meteorite from another planet. And where did that planet get life? It was like the old Indian myth that the earth is upheld by an elephant: the elephant is supported on the back of a great tortoise; and any further question was deprecated as inconvenient curiosity. The discussions on all these matters are too familiar to be pursued further. Our question now is whether we are on the brink of a fourth phase in Evolution Theories, and whether General Smuts is helping to bring that phase any nearer.

Position Before and After Darwin

Our points of inquiry are mainly two. (1) General Smuts claims the right to deal with the whole question without reference to Infinity. Creation *ex nihilo* is to him "unintelligible"; and he considers that the idea of God cannot be inferred from the visible world and may therefore be ignored in a discussion of it. (2) He thinks there are only three "jumps" to be accounted for—matter, life and mind. These two positions of his mark the weak points in his theory, and must be fully discussed before we can safely declare how far we agree with him in the main.

CHAPTER V

CAN THE INFINITE BE IGNORED?

In Catholic philosophy, even when origins are not in question, it is customary to call all finite "causes" secondary. Our very language thus keeps us from losing sight of the First Cause. Is this a necessity of thought, or merely an exercise of devotion? It is, of course, both, for all true thought is based on Absolute Truth, and in Catholic Philosophy truth is always carried into practical exercise. We hold that God Who by His essence is Being itself (or Absolute Being) is therefore intimately present in every finite (or derived) being. And this not only when that being comes into existence, but as long as it is maintained in that existence. God not only creates,

Can the Infinite Be Ignored? 29

but sustains what He has created. "Upholding all things by the word of His power." While, therefore, we agree that Evolution shows a continuous progressive creativeness, we add that this creativeness is nothing else than the effect in time of the original creative and sustaining Word. Those, therefore, who read the book we are reviewing must read into it this relation to the Infinite, for General Smuts does not explicitly put it there.

Our concept of any individual thing is not merely the sum total of our knowledge of its phenomena: an essential part of the concept is its relation to the Absolute. Of course we may use partial concepts for partial purposes. We may in science mark off an investigation into secondary causes alone. But we must always know and remember that such concepts are incomplete. We may in mathematics talk of the limited front of a parabola between the focus and the vertex, and say we have "squared" the parabola as two-thirds of its containing rectangle; but we go wrong if we forget that the centre of the parabola has been projected to infinity. And, whatever we may do in limited fields of science, we must in philosophy deal with *complete* concepts. Now General Smuts is talking philosophy, and is professing to give a complete explanation of Evolution. He must not, therefore, and probably does not intend to, omit its relativity to the Infinite.

It might be asked, What difference does it make to a stone or a plant if I sufficiently sum up its phenomena and omit all reference to the Power that made it and keeps it what it is? Little difference perhaps to the stone or the plant, but a great deal of difference in the attitude of the mind. Continue the habit of ignoring the infinite relation, and in due time you come to consider yourself objectively with the same omission; and for an intellectual being to consider itself as self-subsistent opens wide the door to that pride of mind and will which obscures truth more than anything else in the world.

Can the Infinite Be Ignored?

Towards the end of the book General Smuts does in a way face the question. He says: "There is universal agreement with the well-known argument of Kant, that from the facts of Nature no inference of God is justified." Let him reconsider the word "universal." The whole mass of Catholic Philosophy looks upon this as one of Kant's greatest blunders. Given any sort of finite world and any finite mind to contemplate that world, and a valid inference of Infinitude in Goodness, Truth and Beauty might rush into that mind by every channel of perception. He goes on: "The belief in the Divine Being rests, and necessarily must rest, on quite different grounds." Even so, as soon as a man acquires that belief, no matter whence, it should have its place in his science as well as in his religion. All that we know of God, however we acquire it, necessarily forms part of our concept of any of His work. We should deal with *whole* concepts in philosophy. General Smuts is a Holist and should be consistent.

Our next point will be to consider the gaps that have to be bridged in giving a continuous story of the growth of the universe. Throughout the book General Smuts speaks lightly of the *three* stages "matter, life, mind," and he jumps from one to another without a qualm. We shall have to point out that one of his jumps we may tentatively make with him, though Science has not yet done so; a second we may make on the evidence; but there is a third which we have to declare impossible except to a second creative Word, and a fourth (the greatest of all) which he ignores as not within his ken, though it is well in his field of phenomena.

CHAPTER VI

STAGES OF EVOLUTION

JUST as Catholic Philosophy refuses to consider secondary "causes" without at least an implicit reference to the First Cause, because by so doing it would be dealing with incomplete concepts, so it refuses to omit the purely spiritual world (that of Angels) and still more the supernatural (the Kingdom of Grace) from its explanations of the Universe. These things cannot indeed be put into a chemical or physical laboratory, but materialistic science, marvellous as its processes are and beautiful as its results, is not the only way to truth. And these conceptions are not merely subjective phenomena of religion. It cannot be said that the Resurrection of Jesus Christ is out of touch with the realities of human history, and the World of Grace appeals to as wide an experience as the World of Nature. It seems to be claimed that face to face with sceptical forms of thought we should lay aside not only all Revelation, but also all the experiences that have resulted from Revelation. Whatever we may do when we argue with them, we decline to lay aside sources of our own knowledge when we think for ourselves. The first tempter began with the insinuation, "Yea, hath God said?" But we who know that God hath said are not so tied to the devil's tail that we are to keep on repeating his fallacious old question. When, therefore, we lay down *our* list of the grades of being, it is not that we wish to force our own beliefs on incredulous opponents, but simply that we want to clear our own ideas and find out for ourselves how far it is possible for us, and how far we must refuse, to go step by step with evolution theories.

Moreover, when we make our list, we must remember that we do not know when the world

Stages of Evolution

was created. It may have been just before the appearance of man. At whatever stage the world was created, it was necessarily created with an apparent past history. It must have been formed as if it had always obeyed the laws which henceforth it was to obey. It looks as if it had existed for millions of years, but it would look like that if it was first formed some ten or twenty thousand years ago—fossils and all. We simply do not know. It is as easy for the Infinite Creator to think backward as to think forward. There is no time or succession for God. We therefore look back into the millions of years past "without prejudice." No matter at what stage God created the world, it must have had an apparently illimitable past. It is only the apparent record that we can study.

Further, when our list is made, if we find that the known laws of any stage do not to the best of our knowledge make the next stage possible, there is nothing for it but to suspend our judgment and to say, "Either evolution proceeded by some principle unknown to us, or the First Cause intervened." *Natura non facit saltum,* and we must not either.

These provisos being premised, we may arrange our stages of being somewhat as follows:—

(1) The "primeval fire-mist" (if it ever existed as a stage). It is too indeterminate to make any appeal to our imagination. The thought of it is the nearest we can come to a conception of Aristotle's *materia prima.* It is quite homely beginning thus with the old philosopher.

(2) Atoms, *i.e.* nuclei with varying numbers of electrons (whatever nuclei and electrons are). The present phase of speculation seems to say that the only difference between one atom and another lies in the number of its electrons. Let them have it as they like, but this predominance of mere number would delight old Pythagoras. This little smile does not diminish my admiration for the marvellous

delicacy of measurement, invention and observation by the scientists of our day.

(3) Molecular combination into substances on a big scale, whether gaseous, liquid or solid, in the last case culminating in the regularity and beauty of crystal forms.

(4) Colloid substances which show an uncanny similarity to the processes of life.

(5) Protoplasm, or life-substance, usually at once building cell-walls for its protection. This substance even in its lowest forms shows a responsiveness to outside influences which gives us as a definition of life "a continuous adaptation of internal to external relations." This carries us to the heights of the plant world.

(6) Sense is added to responsiveness, and characterises the whole animal world. Diverse as (5) and (6) are in the higher stages, they are to our perceptions almost indistinguishable in the lower. But our means of perception are very imperfect.

(7) In Man, reason, and therefore spirituality and immortality, is superadded.

(8) Angelic, *i.e.* purely spiritual, beings.

(9) The Kingdom of Grace, in which spiritual beings are participant and material things ministrant, and which consists of the Word made Flesh and the members of His Mystical Body.

With regard to this list, General Smuts of course says nothing about (8) or (9), and for the present we hold them back. What we have to discuss is the question of how to jump from (4) to (5), from (5) to (6), and above all from (6) to (7). Curiously enough, General Smuts discusses the first two of these jumps, but totally ignores the third. He takes three steps—one from the flat to a molehill, one from the molehill to an antheap; the third he quietly assumes lands him on top of Table Mountain. This Munchausen seven-league step requires a good deal of discussion, and that will occupy us next time.

CHAPTER VII

BRIDGING THE GAPS

In the series of stages enumerated last time, the first arguable question comes in the leap from crystalline and colloid structure to protoplasm or life-substance. As we have seen, the old philosophers and the scholastics felt no difficulty here. Indeed, they thought it was a fact of experience that living creatures were spawned out of the teeming slime of rivers and marshes by the energy of the sun. The point is that it did not worry them. Increased knowledge of science, however, brought the maxim *omne vivum ex vivo*. A spontaneous origin for life has not yet been observed, though it has been very eagerly sought for. General Smuts puts the origin millions of years ago when conditions were more favourable. "It is not improbable," he says in one of the admirable summaries prefixed to his chapters, "that the cell of life arose when the sun was both warmer and richer in chemically active rays, and when the waters of the earth still contained many substances in solution and colloid dispersal." This gives us a somewhat hypothetical probability. The point, however, is not of practical importance in this discussion. It is merely a question of whether we shall say that there are two evolutions or one. I do not understand the importance that some of our philosophers attribute to the necessity of "special creation" of the first germs. I see no reason why spontaneous origins of life should not be going on even now. Nature's laboratory is much better equipped than the scientist's. In watching an amœba, which seems to be nothing but undifferentiated protoplasm without even a cell wall, I find it hard to believe that in a world of perpetual change this little thing has been able to maintain its simplicity by mere division for millions of years. Of course it may be a degenerate form; but, as far as I know, degenerate forms always contain rudiments of the forms from which they have come down. Yeast, for example, by budding instead of merely dividing, retains an absurd little resemblance to the higher alga forms from which it is thought to have deteriorated. At any rate it would cause me no surprise if a spontaneous emergence of life were discovered to-morrow. If it should be, I only hope it will not be under such conditions as to put the control of it in the hands of the discoverer. It is easier to upset the balance of Nature than to readjust it, and a breeder of spontaneous germs might introduce appalling pestilences into the world.

The gap between the vegetative and the sensitive life is very great when we compare higher forms only; but in the lower grades it is sometimes hard to distinguish plant from animal. The amœba, which is classed as an animal, seems distinctly lower than the diatom, which is undoubtedly a plant. But as our philosophers hold that the souls (or "forms") of both plants and animals are "educed from the potentiality of matter," it does not seem difficult to grant that evolution may have been continuous from the chaotic state up to the animal world. If it should hereafter be proved that the laws of inorganic matter can never suffice to produce a living germ, and if it should be proved that plant laws can never of themselves rise to sense, then we should have to say that the original Creative Word (as far as matter is concerned) was threefold: (1) let there be matter; (2) when certain conditions are reached, let there be life; (3) when further conditions are reached, let there be sensation. But as these two propositions seem not likely ever to be proved, we may well incline to the belief that the *fiats* (2) and (3) are not really distinct from (1). St. Augustine would say that we should be postulating miracles, and miracles are not to be expected at that stage.

The step from Sense to Intellect is a very different matter. The world's greatest thinkers have maintained that, under the controlling laws, sense-life could not possibly be evolved into thought-life. Consequently the origin of the spirit-soul of man must be co-ordinated with that of the Angels.

Of course, General Smuts says nothing about Angels: he would place them outside normal experience. But the extraordinary thing is that he (apparently in complete unconsciousness) *assumes* without discussion as an axiom what the majority of the greatest philosophers strongly deny. As soon as he comes to Sensation he calls it "Mind." His constant division is Matter, Life, Mind. With him the mind of man differs only in degree from the mind of a dog. Let us be logical at least. Why stop at the dog? Other stages, differing only in degree, are the canary, the lizard, the snail, the flea, the worm, right down to the amoeba. Are these all intellectual and spiritual?

Many anecdotes (frequently told with a bias) represent animals, especially dogs, as "thinking." I am much interested in these, and out of the thousands I have read or been told there is not one that cannot easily be explained by sense or instinct. We often hear of dogs baying the moon, but we have never heard of a dog trying to classify or enumerate the stars. This is a "popular" rather than a scientific or philosophic difficulty; so we must give it a sort of "popular" solution. Sentimental women who are sure of the immortality of their pet Pom do not need answering; but there are scientists, supposedly sane, who are (with undisguised bias) trying to prove the intellectuality of dogs and monkeys. At the risk of being overwhelmed with protests and "proofs," I will deal with this matter next time.

CHAPTER VIII

SENSE AND REASON

THE sciences of Biology and Psychology are deplorably indeterminate as to their common boundaries, and even as to their common domains. This uncertainty is a measure of the harm done to clear thinking by the mechanistic theories of Descartes. In spite of the second half of the two words (-logy) there is not much logic in their arrangement. Biology breaks up into Botany and Zoology. If the whole life and soul of the oak is treated under Botany, why is not the whole life and soul of the dog treated under Zoology? If, on the other hand, the soul (*psyche*) of the dog is treated under Psychology, why not also the soul (*psyche*) of the oak? The psychological difference between the oak and the dog is small compared to that between the dog and the man.

The fact is that, tempted by the apparent easiness of it, scientists endeavour to explain the whole *psyche* of the plant in terms of mechanical and chemical processes. They then link the *psyche* of the animal to that of the man. The third process would be to bring the animals down to the plant-level, dragging humanity with them. Didn't the nineteenth century promise us an *homunculus* in a laboratory bottle? Didn't Goethe put it on the stage?

But in truth they cannot explain even the mechanical processes of the plant. How does a lofty tree raise the sap through open vessels up some 300 or 400 feet? Add together the root pressure, and the lift of liquid in minute tubes, and ingenious arrangements of pumping, and they fall short of even 100 feet. As General Smuts says, the combination is always more than the sum of the parts.

Now note that some plants are able to mock the higher processes of animals. The sensitive plant and the sundews act absurdly as if they had nerves. But there is not the smallest reason to suppose that the sensitive plant (*Mimosa pudica*) is more highly organised than other mimosas; and it is certainly below the daisy in development. In a similar way some animals have uncanny ways of apparently anticipating intellectual processes. The bower-bird (whose antics, however, have been much coloured by bias) seems to be capable of æsthetic delight. It turns out to be merely an appetite for bright things, as with the magpie and the ostrich. There is no reason for putting the bower-bird nearer to humanity than the peacock.

In most cases, however, of apparently rational actions in animals we are dealing with domesticated varieties. Their cleverness is merely a reflection or imitation of their master's ways. We mesmerise our pets. On this account, marks of "intelligence" should be sought for only in wild creatures. There is a scientist now who employs himself in setting problems to apes. They solve these problems.

Of course: they see he wants them to do something; they try one thing after another; they see indications which he is not conscious of showing; and all the time they only want to do what he expects for the sake of the reward. It is clever, but the man has missed his vocation: he is thrown away on a science room: he should be in a circus.

The stock proof of a dog's logic seems to me to prove the very opposite. They say that a dog following a trail came to where three roads diverged. He smelt along one and came back. Then he smelt along the second and failed again. The third time he went unhesitatingly down the third road without smelling his way at all. Now it seems to me that a thinking dog would first find out in which direction the scent was strongest before twice making a fool of himself by running down false trails. He took the third road without hesitation, not because he could argue from logical premises, but because the scent was there and his nose told him so.

Sense and Reason

It must be remembered that in all the senses we are surpassed by one or other of the animals, some of them seeming to have senses denied to us. Moreover, instinct can in some respects even surpass reason in small matters. We, for example, should never have thought of, or been able to perform, the wonderful feat of the ichneumon wasp, which paralyses every separate nerve centre of a caterpillar except one, and then injures that one, so as to have a living but helpless prey for a future brood of grubs. Evolution is very far indeed from being able to explain even so simple a case as that.

While, therefore, we have the power of soaring to the heights of non-material thought, we also know that included in our being are all the animal tendencies, all the vegetative growth, all chemical combinations, all mechanical forces. Because they are within us, we are able to measure them one against another; and we know that all our lower powers together have it not in the laws of their structure ever to rise to the height of thought. We know then that our soul is a *psyche* indeed, but immensely more than a *psyche*. It is this knowledge that assures us of spirituality and consequent immortality.

CHAPTER IX

THE THREEFOLD CREATIVE WORD

HITHERTO I have been considering not what General Smuts has expressly put forward as his theory, but what the Catholic student should have in his own mind while studying that theory. I fully believe that a great deal of what I have been "reading into" this book is implicitly contained therein; and I want Catholic students to read it from that point of view. It is not a usual point of view. That is to say, General Smuts, writing for scientists and natural philosophers, is silent on certain topics, and in our ordinary experience such silence usually indicates antagonism. It is not so here. The aim of the whole book is spiritual, not materialistic.

Let me, therefore, before positively expounding what Holism is, state very concisely the view of Creation and Evolution which seems to me most consistent with Catholic Philosophy.

The Creative Word, which put forth this universe in all its complexity and liberty is in itself absolutely One. But for us, creatures of time, space and contingency, this oneness is not within our ken. It is like the light of the sun, which is most useful to us in the normal diffusion of daylight, most beautiful in the refraction of the rainbow and the diffraction of iridescence, most instructive in its threefold division of Light, Heat and Actinism.

Of these three aspects, the best is the childlike way of attributing everything directly to Our Heavenly Father—an attitude which Christ Our Lord approved above everything else. The second is the way of poets and artists. The third is the way of philosophy—not essential for all, but necessary because men *will* think.

We may say then that the Creative Word is refracted for us into three *fiats*: (1) Let there be matter, with all its potentialities of order and organic life; (2) Let there be spiritual beings, some purely so, some with the power of animating matter; (3) Let there be a power (Grace) lifting these things to the Divine. Fitly, therefore, does the song of Creation begin with "Let there be Light"—the light of the vision of the Universe, the light of the vision of Truth, and the light of the vision of God.

St. Augustine, expounding this view, seems to say (and with this, of course, the Church does not agree), that along with the Angels at the beginning all souls of men were also created ready to be breathed into their material envelope when their time should come. The idea, so expressed, was Platonic, and Wordsworth has made us familiar with it. But I feel sure that St. Augustine meant no substantial preexistence (in our sense of *pre-*) for individual souls. His faith-instincts were far too deep and keen to make him an uncertain guide in matters so fundamental. His meaning surely is that the creation of each human soul is (1) direct, but not (2) miraculous. It is direct because virtually contained in the second Creative Word: it is not miraculous because it proceeds from the normal laws of that Word.

As a parallel illustration, the change at the moment of consecration in the Mass is God's direct action from the third Creative Word, but not (ordinarily speaking) miraculous because it is in accordance with the normal laws of that Word. Of course from the plane of Nature it is full of miracle, and in a similar way the creation of a human soul is in the natural order of the second Word, but a marvel from the plane of matter.

Our path is now clear before us to expound what Holism is. The word is unfamiliar, but it will soon become well enough known. As I have already intimated, it is closely akin to what our philosophy has called "substantial forms," but both "substance" and "form" have been so misused in the history of thought that a new word is quite welcome.

CHAPTER X

WHAT IS HOLISM?

It is about time I answered this question after talking about Holism through nine chapters. But I wanted my Catholic readers to get a firm grip on the right point of view before positively expounding the theory. The word is from the Greek *holos,* whole, and might be written Wholism, except that scientific terms are generally taken from Latin or Greek so as to be internationally intelligible. The reason for the name will appear at once.

Let us first take a simple, though inadequate, analogy. Two boys have each a good Meccano set, and they are asked to give their views on it. One describes enthusiastically all the contents of the box, the parts, the wheels, the nuts, etc., and shows how he keeps them all complete and unspoiled, without caring very much what he makes out of his play. The other is excited about the crane, the motor-car, the donkey-engine, etc., already to his credit, and talks hopefully about making something that nobody has yet seen. The first boy takes a Mechanistic view of his set; the second an Holistic view.

So two scientists are face to face with the visible world. One thinks of breaking it up to see what it is made of. Complex substances he analyses into simpler ones, largely ignoring what he may be losing in the analytical process. At last he comes to the irreducible elements, and is able to announce that all material things are composed of some ninety odd of them. Not satisfied with that, he goes on to break up even the atoms and finds that (instead of the indivisible, indestructible minima of last century) they are little "solar systems," consisting of positively electrified nuclei with one or two or many negative electrons dancing round them.

Thus he looks upon the universe as made up of nuclei (of which he confesses he knows but little) and electrons (of which he claims to know that they are all exactly alike)—and nothing else. This is only saying on the big scale what he says on the small: *e.g.* a molecule of water is just two atoms of hydrogen combined with one of oxygen—and nothing else. Thus he has totality divided into its ultimate parts which can be mentally reassembled, into the huge world-machine wound up ready to go.

This, somewhat baldly stated, is the Mechanistic view. But observe that I am not in any way belittling the analytic process. It is not only necessary, but its rapidly accelerating skill and efficiency fills us with admiration. The apparatus, for example, which makes visible to the naked eye the path of a single helium atom exploding from radium is perhaps the most effective demonstration in the whole range of physical teaching. It is not the positive analysis we object to, but the implied assumption "and nothing more." It is the

What is Holism? 59

ignoring of what may have been lost in the analysis.

The other scientist is the Holist. He takes full cognisance, with equal delight, of the skilful work of the Analyst; but he says to him: "You must have left something out, something which your laboratory tests do not touch, but which Nature reveals. You take protoplasm from the dead body of a cat and from the dead body of a man, and you say that in both cases it is chemically a very complex substance, but that you can still give all the parts of it, and your analysis makes the two protoplasms the same. Something has been left out, for the life of man is much higher than the life of a cat, and in both cases it is the protoplasm that carries the life." Then he goes to the base of things, fixing his mind on the "something more." Starting with the atom he would say that an isolated nucleus (could such a thing be found) and a stray electron are barren by themselves, but put them together and you get an atom of hydrogen, a new substance: they have "created" something. So an atom of oxygen is greatly more than a nucleus *plus* eight electrons. So through the elements. In the next stage two wandering atoms of hydrogen meet an atom of oxygen, each with definite properties of its own: somehow the three of them fuse into an entirely new substance: they have "created" water. And important as oxygen is, they have gone higher than themselves, for water is the matrix of life. Then some carbon atoms come strolling along and join with water, and something new is formed, something more than $C + H + O$, and more important because the carbohydrates are the main food of life. And so the creative series goes on, with ever more freedom, more complexity, more delicacy until the range of human life is reached.

The Holist would explain: "I do not need now to say whence matter got its creativeness. I see a continuous chain from Chaos to Spirituality. If and when intervention from the Infinite has been necessary, that intervention has not broken the continuity of the chain. It has only emphasized the fact that even the material world is always groaning and travailing after the liberty and idealism of the spiritual."

I must leave my readers to see for themselves how General Smuts has unfolded this thesis in chapter after chapter of a book as remarkable for scientific breadth as for lucid expression. There is still much to say. I have yet to compare these "wholes" with the Aristotelian and scholastic "forms." I have to question the accuracy of making the Cell the unit of life as the Atom is the unit of inorganic matter. I have to answer some *obiter dicta* about Catholic morality. I intend to have a little scrap with the Theory of Relativity. And above all I must point to the supreme Totum or Whole which is the ultimate reason and goal of all those that have preceded.

CHAPTER XI

IS THE CELL THE UNIT OF ORGANIC LIFE?

It is no wonder that the cell has often been chosen as the unit of life. First of all there are the countless myriads of unicellular organisms. Microscopic as they are, they are of immense importance in the mass. Of diatoms alone, in which Nature seems to be trying the experiment how much variety of beauty of form she can throw into a speck of matter, we can say that under our direct observation they are building up geological strata with their tiny flinty skeletons. Secondly, all the higher organisms pass twice through a unicellular stage. Every single living cell is a marvellous little world of its own, but the reproductive cells baffle our research and stagger the imagination.

Thirdly, under the microscope all the higher organisms *seem* to be aggregations of cells, each of which has an independent life of its own, while yet they co-operate towards the completer life of the whole. I underline the word *seems,* because further investigation shows that the appearance is not quite in accordance with fact. Mechanistic scientists are anxious that we should accept this theory of an aggregation. Nay, General Smuts himself seems to accept it, and explains the unity of the totum by each cell being in the "field" of its neighbours' activities. But I question the word "aggregation": the cells are not aggregated because they never were segregated. I do not say that any scientists want to conceal the truth, but they do not see the force of what they themselves have with marvellous skill demonstrated. I will return to this point. These three considerations give great colour to the theory that the cell is the unit of life.

But there are other considerations. First of all there are very simple forms that are not cellular. The amœba has no more cell-wall than a drop of oil: it completely changes its shape from moment to moment according to its requirements. Sometimes such unclothed masses of protoplasm form themselves into colonies (plasmodia), the individuals being separable but not separated; and in this case they are true aggregations, of which the unit is a single little mass of protoplasm. Secondly, there are many seaweeds which find the water-support sufficient and do not build internal cell-walls at all, such as Caulerpa, etc. In the growth of such plants the nuclei divide and separate but are still held together by strands of streaming protoplasm. Some botanists call such a plant unicellular, but this is surely a misnomer. It should be called, what it really is, a multi-nuclear mass of protoplasm surrounded by a wall. This external wall is different in both function and origin from the usual internal cell-walls. Even in the really unicellular plants it is different. If you have one under observation through the microscope (Volvox I sup-

Is Cell Unit of Organic Life? 65

pose would do, and it is fairly big), you can run a solution of salt under the cover-glass and draw it through with a bit of blotting-paper. As soon as the salt touches the cell-wall, all the protoplasm standing on guard at that wall shrinks away from it and retreats as if for protection on to the nucleus. If you allow the salt solution to penetrate the wall by physical osmosis, you kill the protoplasm. But if you reverse the current at once, draw away the salt and let fresh water return, the protoplasm goes back to its sentry duty and the whole plant seems as happy as before. This could not take place in an internal cell. The life-substance could not leave the cell-wall without lesion.

Thirdly, consider the normal mode of growth. A single cell has its walls lengthened: the nucleus breaks up into two, and the halves separate with quaint ceremonies of a fairy dance but remain united by many protoplasmic strands which arrange themselves in the form of a spindle. While the half-nuclei grow to their full size, they build up a wall, or rather two walls, between them, until the one cell has become completely two. But the spindle-shaped cluster of life threads remains, and indeed persists throughout the life of that part of the plant. The cell-wall is pierced with little tunnels through which the life-substance of each cell is in continuous communication with that of its neighbour. It is like the many-arched wall of the Coliseum through which the Romans of old poured in and out as easily as if it were all gate. This continuum has been beautifully shown in a mature leaf of the oleander (Nerium). The protoplasm was first paralysed, then killed. Then the section was treated with an acid which should dissolve the cell-walls without acting on the dead protoplasm. The section was then cleaned and stained. The result was a delicate lace-like pattern of unbroken threads, dead now but formerly the very life of the oleander leaf.

There is an Indian botanist, whose imagination seems to have overcome his undoubtedly great intellect, who chloroforms plants, and talks of their nerves and measures their heart-beats. His facts are correct, and he marshals them skilfully, but his deductions are not valid. There is nothing new to us in the fact that protoplasm (life) can be poisoned. It does not need nerves to explain the widely extended response to stimulus: it only needs continuity. All life-processes are rhythmic, and therefore they can be rhythmically recorded; but to talk of a heart, say in a mushroom, is sheer non-sense. If this gentleman goes on like that, one of these days a dandelion will deliberately make a long nose at him. But, as I said, his facts are correct, and what they do is to give a physiological proof of what we know otherwise, that the protoplasm is continuous throughout the plant.

This is a marvellous conception. It is not to the point to say that the protoplasmic threads (I am sorry for the ungainly word: life-threads, if you will) are very attenuated, almost ultramicroscopic in their thinness. A square yard of lace, however filmy, is just as much a continuous textile fabric as a yard of brocade. So, with this conception in our mind, let us look at an oak tree. What we touch and see in the oak is (with one exception) not the oak itself but the glorious mansion it has built for itself—the external walls for protection and the internal ones for support and accommodation. The one exception is the green colour of the leaves and young stems. This green is the colour of the chlorophyll grains, the structure which provides the food of the world. General Smuts calls chlorophyll a colloidal substance; but it is far higher, it is protoplasmic. Colloids are so called because they are like glue, though above it. Chlorophyll then might be called colloidoidal, because it is like colloids, though above them. The green colour therefore shows us the real oak-life shining out of the windows of its palace and beautifying the world.

Now, looking at the oak tree as a whole, think away all the structure of walls, and you see a vast and continuous mass of protoplasm, fairy-like in its daintiness of branching form, so delicate that a breath would injure it, yet braving the storms of centuries and providing the world with a very type of strength and endurance. It is a single totality, a totum, a whole. The oak is its own unity just as much as is the pleurococcus or the amœba.

There are exceptional cells, *e.g.* spermatozoa, blood corpuscles, etc. But they are life-carriers, and do not really break the unity.

This self-contained unity is nowhere better shown than in the autumnal leaf-fall. Many people think that the cold weather kills the leaves, and the oak takes a winter rest to recover from the weakening shock. The truth is quite contrary to this. If a twig is killed, not only will the leaves not fall off, it will require a strong effort to pull them off. What happens is this. On the approach of cold weather, all the protoplasm in the leaves organises a strategic retreat "according to plan." The baggage, the useful commissariat, is sent down into the stem to be stored. The protoplasm evacuates cell after cell and retreats to the stem line ready fortified for it, just like Wellington's great withdrawal within the lines of Torres Vedras. While the fortification line is being completed, afterwards seen as the leaf-scar, a little of the protoplasm is left outside to build up a separation-layer of thin-walled cells between the abandoned leaf form and the stem, and when that is done it retires into shelter, closes up its line of retreat, and waits for the first stiff breeze to blow away the now-useless outhouse. So far from the life of the oak being weakened by shock, it is concentrated into fuller strength, having also conserved its wealth of storage. It goes into winter quarters and rests with nothing to disturb it but the holiday task of solidifying its timber. And therein lies the explanation of the annual miracle of the spring revival.

I therefore maintain that each plant is a unit in itself, and by parallel argument each animal also: that therefore the biological unit is not "the cell" but "a continuous mass of protoplasm." I suggest this idea to General Smuts as being far more in accordance with his theory of Holism than that of a mere aggregation of separate cells which are not separate.

CHAPTER XII

"WHOLES" AND "SUBSTANTIAL FORMS"

How Aristotle and the Scholastics would have modified their theory of Matter and Form if they had known the results of modern analysis it would be idle to discuss. In practice the distinction is perceptible only by intellect and is hardly expressible in words. Science has now resolved all the tangible universe into atoms of some ninety different kinds. It, moreover, now claims to have resolved all atoms into nuclei and electrons. Further, they suspect that these electrons (and I suppose nuclei also) are nothing but vortices of the ether which we are obliged to postulate as a medium for the transmission of waves of light and other "forces." That is to say, they have reduced all matter to a basic indefinable substance indefinitely varied by forces playing upon it. Their formula then is that the visible world is equal to ether *plus* combinations of forces (which make wholes or forms). Aristotle's would be that the visible world is equal to *materia prima* plus its moulding forces. He would say: "Your formula is only one step in front of mine, for your ether is equal to *materia prima* plus the one form of capacity for transmitting force."

There has of late been a rebellion against the victorious ether, and General Smuts takes up a doubtful stand. But if this ether is dethroned, we shall have to substitute for it another vague substance with exactly the same quality of elasticity; and we may as well call the new substance by the same name. In that case the difference of ultimate basis between Lord Kelvin and Aristotle becomes very filmy. I wrote a paper on the subject in the *Dublin Review* many years ago, but I never heard if anybody read it besides the printers. At that time my paper, originally read for the Royal

Society of S. Africa, was pooh-poohed as "metaphysics." But medievalism is coming into its own. *Materia prima* is just as much science as ether is.

To show again that these are no new thoughts with me, I treated the whole theory twenty-five years ago in a book (now out of print) called *The Art of Life*. One paragraph in it was headed "The almost-nothingness of matter and the everythingness of the form," and the concept was applied to man's nature in the words: "This body of ours is not a separate thing, different from the soul. We deny that it has any organic life of its own which a super-added soul comes in by some mysterious influence to control and direct. Sensation is not a gathering by the soul of impressions on particles united to but external to itself. The body has not even a being it can call its own: whatever the body is, the soul makes it. The moving of the limbs, the circulation of the blood, the renovation of tissue, the digestion of food, are all as much the work of the soul as are sensation and thought. I am one being, not two. My soul is simple in its essence, as well as various in its powers; and it is one and the same thing which thinks beyond the body's range, which in the body feels, which organises the body itself, and which constitutes (or gives being to) the very minutest particle of which that body is composed." All this is included in the meaning of the statement that "the soul is the *form* of the body!" Every human being is a unique *totum* or whole, a single substantial form with its basic matter.

And the whole is not merely the sum of the parts. Nor is it anything superadded to the parts. It *is* the parts in their co-existence and co-activities. This General Smuts says over and over again almost in the words of St. Thomas Aquinas himself. To give just one sentence: "Forma substantialis totius non superadditur partibus, sed est totum complectens materiam et formam cum præcisione aliorum."

It is the clearness with which General

Smuts has seen this, the wealth of illustration he has devoted to it, and the consequences he has drawn from it, that give the value to this work on *Holism and Evolution*. When it was first announced that General Smuts had a work on philosophy in preparation, I ventured to approach him with a suggestion of preliminary discussion. He told me, however, that it was already in the hands of the printers, adding with a whimsical smile: "I will send you a copy, and then you can tell me where I am wrong." It has been to me a great surprise, and a much greater pleasure, to find so much in which I can tell him where he is right.

CHAPTER XIII

THE THEORY OF RELATIVITY

WHILE urging us to reform our concepts of matter, space, time, etc., General Smuts expounds with vivacity and enthusiasm Einstein's Theory of Relativity. This theory has been ushered into the world with a great flourish of trumpets, and claims have been made for it which must make Einstein shudder. I have seen it stated that a man measured one way might be 6 ft. 3 in. in height, and another way 4 ft. 6 in., and that he does not notice these remarkable changes because everything around changes with him. Any practical difference of measurement due to Relativity will be somewhere near the 10th decimal place when we think in inches. If a farmer, hearing that

78 A Catholic View of Holism

"Euclid's geometry no longer holds" and that "Newton's laws of motion are scrapped," were to come to me in anxiety about the value of his farm, I should take a penny and ask him to divide it mentally into 1,000 parts; then to divide each of those thousandths also into 1,000 parts; one of these last microscopic portions would be about the difference in value that Einstein's Theory (if it were proved) would make to his farm in about 100 years. Einstein himself says there is no test for his valuations except in the stellar spaces. There he has two scores to his credit—(1) some eccentricities in the planet Mercury, and (2) the bending of a ray of light passing the face of the sun. But on earth the theory makes no practical difference and cannot be of any use for Holism.

Some of the "facts" which General Smuts adduces will hardly hold. For example, he states that if there is a sudden flash of light, and there are two persons, one standing beside it and one speeding away from it at half the velocity of light, the flash will be simul-

The Theory of Relativity 79

taneously visible to both of them. It is very easy to make such imaginary experiments. It is equally easy to deny them; and this I do deny. It is impossible for a sentient being to travel at half the speed of light. But make it sound instead of light, and daily experience tells us that the experiment would fail.

Then there is Einstein's "cage." He imagines a person enclosed in a cage and put in a non-gravitational region. Then he imagines another "force" acting on this cage causing accelerated motion. Then he guesses what would happen to the person inside the cage. What can anybody prove by such unreal experiments? What does he know of gravitation more than anybody else? Would an organic body even hold together without gravity? How could this body in the cage have any "weight" if there were no gravity? General Smuts thinks Einstein's cage will be as historical as Newton's apple. I think it will be remembered only as a joke. Nothing, whether in science, or mathematics, or philosophy, has any proving value unless we keep our feet on *terra firma*. We can't get outside of ourselves.

Here a critic may severely ask me how I dare to laugh at so supreme an authority in Physics and Mathematics. I do not laugh at him in his own line. Far from it. *Cuique in arte sua credendum.* But a mathematician is not necessarily an authority, say, in music. All men have their limitations. Descartes was a supreme mathematician, but all his philosophy has crumbled into ineptitude. W. K. Clifford was a first-rate physicist and mathematician, but he made us laugh when he tried to imagine a one-dimension universe, taking as his imaginary experiment an intellectual worm in a tube which he just fitted. Unless that worm was merely one of Euclid's abstract lines, he would have the three dimensions in himself. He would have at least the worm-like attribute of being able to wriggle; and like the proverbial worm he might try to turn. He could push upwards and downwards, to right and to left, and could move forwards and backwards, and where

The Theory of Relativity 81

is your one-dimensional universe? In other words, Clifford trying to imagine himself an intellectual worm was only making a jackass of himself. I refuse to be bluffed by revolutionary speculators.

The fact is that mathematicians, besides the pitfalls which philosophy offers to all men, are peculiarly liable to be misled by their own symbols, and the more their symbolic skill the greater is their danger. The operation of algebraical symbols is wider than the range of reality. To take a very simple instance, I solve the following problem:—"What are eggs a dozen when two more in a shilling's-worth lowers the price one penny per dozen?" I find at once that the answer is 9d. a dozen. But the same symbolic equation gives me the foolish answer *minus* 8d. The second answer has a meaning, but this can only be understood by reinterpreting my symbols in terms of common fact. In other words, the results of symbolic calculations must always be retranslated into solid fact before they can be trusted. You cannot get out of an equation more than you have put into it. When, therefore, Einstein writes down a result of calculation in one of his fearsome differential equations, and then triumphantly says, "This proves that the universe is finite," I say, "No, my dear sir; it only proves that your arbitrary symbols are applicable only to a finite part of the universe: total reality is not subject to symbols." Of course the universe is finite: if it were not, it would be God; but that is not to say that we are so constituted as to be able to fathom its finitude.

We may well, therefore, pause before we upset our useful old geometry and the laws of motion. These are mental abstractions, and will endure as long as mind endures. You may add to them, but you cannot upset them. Indeed, what else does Einstein himself say when he declares that Space is curved (whatever he means by that most unphilosophical statement)? To call a thing curved, you must say it is "not straight"; but what does he mean if his theory has upset the idea of "straight"?

The Theory of Relativity 83

Einstein was invited once to Oxford or Cambridge to expound his theory. He had an audience of the foremost mathematicians in England. I am told that the impression he made on the learned Dons was that he did not understand the theory himself.

Fortunately, in the rest of the book General Smuts does not trouble himself with any application of the theory, and Evolution proceeds in the "Space-Time Continuum" only in the sense of our familiar old Space and Time.

CHAPTER XIV

THE MORAL ASPECT OF HOLISM

GENERAL SMUTS is so intent on the higher levels which matter is "creating," which are educible from matter and to which matter is capable of being elevated, that he almost entirely ignores the other side of the process. Matter is not only creative, it is also destructive and (what is worse) self-destructive. As soon as it reaches life it begins to die. As soon as it reaches spirituality it tries to materialise the spiritual. This is a world of Upward and Downward, and we are in it. The moral value of life is to assist the Upward and to resist the Downward, and, carried to its highest point, to love the Life and to hate the Corruption. When around us we see young things dancing for the sheer joy of life's abundance, we rejoice with them: we love the very bodies of innocent children, and our love is without alloy. But when we see and smell the corruption of a corpse we loathe it. Christian philosophy, to which General Smuts has come so near with his Holism, is more holistic than himself. It makes no separation between body and soul: it loves the soul in the body, and the body in the soul. But because both body and soul have their downward as well as their upward trend, it opposes to the body's natural love of mere pleasure the high ideal of purity as revealed in the sacred Body of Christ, and to the soul's natural selfishness of pride the supernatural attitude of humility and obedience. Both mean discipline, and discipline means self-denial and mortification. Is this hatred or contempt? Does the farmer hate his vines when he tops off their lovely spring branches that want merely to climb? Does the mother hate her child when she disciplines its little rebellions? Discipline is almost the first word in the social scheme of Christianity. "For the rest, brethren, whatsoever things are true, whatsoever modest, whatsoever just, whatsoever holy, whatsoever lovely, whatsoever of good fame, if there be any virtue, if any praise of *discipline,* think on these things."

With these principles in view, it is most disappointing that General Smuts has in two pages travestied the whole course of Christian asceticism—contrasting it unfavourably with Greek Paganism and even with the licence of the Renaissance. He writes: "The natural and proper tendency is to look upon the body as clean and wholesome, to rejoice in it as something good and beautiful, to make it twin-sister of the spirit and the embodiment of joyousness and wholesome pleasure. That view of the body finds characteristic expression in Greek literature. It may be a Pagan view, but in reality it is the human and true view. It led to respect and reverence for the body, and the culture of the body as a worthy companion of the spirit." That is the sort of one-sided thing

The Moral Aspect of Holism 87

Ruskin used to say. What is the whole truth? Historically, that Greek culture led to the most appalling sink of moral iniquity ever known in the world. Read St. Paul's sketch of it. A social system which compelled young girls, who anywhere else would be reverenced for virginal purity, to prostitute themselves in the temple of Aphrodite as a preliminary to marriage, cannot be said to have "reverenced" the body. Contrast that with the system of mortification and contempt of material things, which produced that galaxy of noble and lovely girls who died rather than give up either faith or their virginity—Margaret, Lucy, Agatha, Catherine, Agnes, "whose names are five sweet symphonies." General Smuts can surely not have thought this matter out.

The next point is that "base superstitions of the East" infected even Christianity, and "medieval civilisation succumbed to and accentuated this horror of the flesh; the monastic ideal with its monkish practices and morbid celibacies bears eloquent testimony to the great fall of the body." Why monkish? Catholics do not talk of parsonish or predikantish. Why morbid? Why celibacies in the plural? There is only one celibacy in Christendom, and it is the celibacy of Our Lord Himself and of St. John the Baptist and of St. Paul and of thousands of the noblest personalities this world has ever known—not morbid, but vivid and vivifying. It is the determination to devote oneself body and soul to the Divine Ideal. So far from degrading the body it lifts all the bodily energies to the spiritual plane. The monastic ideal, what was it? Has General Smuts ever read Montalembert's *Monks of the West*? Let him go to some of our "monastic" missions here in South Africa—say Chishawasha in Rhodesia, Lourdes in Griqualand East, Mariannhill in Natal. What is their purpose? Now, as in the Middle Ages, it is to civilise barbaric peoples by Agriculture and Sanctity. General Smuts is a farmer: does he think Agriculture is the work of a body despised and bullied into weakness? Is it not

The Moral Aspect of Holism 89

essentially the work of a body trained to effective condition by temperance and hard work —along with sanctity the highest exercise of the Greek ideal of *mens sana in corpore sano*?

What he really refers to is the Oriental idea of a dual principle in the world, good and evil —matter being the evil one. This, under the form of Manicheism, infected Christianity only by producing a heresy, a heresy which brought out only more strongly the Catholic teaching that nothing is evil which God created. There was a sort of recrudescence of Manicheism in later times, which explained the Fall of Man as a total corruption of his nature, body and soul. But that is not Catholic: it is Lutheran and Calvinist.

But, perhaps it may be asked, are there not stories of extraordinary penitential practices in the lives of the Saints? There certainly are. There have been abnormal times and conditions. And there have been extraordinary men. And the Catholic Church has always stood for individual moral liberty. The phenomenon is an interesting one and deserves an article to itself. But for normal life the Catholic keynote is gladness for body and soul. England was "Merry England" in the Middle Ages. There are more Feasts than Fasts in the Catholic calendar, and the fasts are by no means severe. And they are tempered when necessary by dispensation. And always and everywhere mortification is guided by humility and obedience, and is under the essential rule of Common Sense. The Catholic Religion is the only one that has lifted Common Sense to the rank of a first principle.

Next time we shall discuss such cases as may be called abnormal—things, as they say, "to be admired but not imitated." Meantime we may express the hope that in a second edition p. 265 may be rewritten, for as it stands it is not worthy of its 344 companions.

CHAPTER XV

EXTREME CASES

EVERY widespread and deep-rooted system of life, besides its normal average, has its maxima and minima; and these must be judged by the laws of the system in which they occur. It is not fair to criticise a Buddhist monk by measures applicable only to an English curate. Even an Indian fakir is not as foolish as he looks to a casual European tourist. If we condemn anybody we must know why we do so. It would not be just to mock at the "monkish practices and morbid celibacies" of Buddhists without an enlightened knowledge of what they have to say for themselves. And the Catholic Church is on a far higher plane.

For the Catholic religion has developed a

complete philosophy for itself, and it is the only one that has done so—a philosophy intellectual, physical, moral, practical, spiritual and mystical. It has pooled all its resources and brings them all to bear on every problem, from the marvels of sanctity to the simple devotions of childhood. For it, mortification is like the physical drill of the spiritual life, and it expects exercises from a Hercules very different from those of a schoolboy. With Our Lord, it likens mortification to the process of pruning, and the pruning given to an olive tree would kill any other tree on the farm. It always tests forms of life, especially mortifications, which seem to be unusual or excessive. This testing is a duty laid upon the bishop of the place, for the faithful must not be misled by false ideals. And these are some of the principles of the test: (1) there must be the right faith (any taint of Manicheism would condemn it at once); (2) it must be based on right reason, *i.e.* in accordance with the laws of human physiology and psychology (*e.g.* it must not

Extreme Cases

mutilate or disable the life; (3) it must be prudent, *i.e.* within the man's powers and with competent counsel taken; (4) it must be proportioned to the other virtues (much penance and little prayer or little charity would never do); (5) it must have the right motives (such as spiritual progress for self and salvation for others); (6) it must be sacrificial (a giving up of lower pleasures or comforts for higher spiritual ends); (7) the intention must be right (union with the Supreme Sacrifice which redeems the world); (8) it must be edifying, and not shocking (regard had to its own time and place); (9) it must be free from spiritual pride; (10) this freedom from pride must be shown by the ultimate test of obedience.

Now let us compare two extreme cases—one that of St. Simeon Stylites (perhaps the very extremest in the story of Christendom) spending his life on a small platform raised high in air by a pillar, and one that of an Indian fakir who has kept his hand closed till the nails have grown right through the flesh or who has kept an arm in one position till the muscles are atrophied. There is no doubt that a superficial judgment would put the two cases on precisely the same level—a marvellous but worse than useless waste of precious human energy. But we have no right to be superficial. Let us apply the tests. If Europeans have told us right about the fakirs (though I suspect a Brahmin would tell it somewhat differently), almost all the ten tests would fail. Whereas St. Simeon comes through all the ten trimphantly.

At the age of sixteen he entered a monastery, but already, with a body extraordinarily adapted to endurance and a soul eager for the heights of mysticism, his austerities went so far beyond the usual that the superiors had to tell him that his mode of life was not proportioned to the community rules. They did not forbid or restrain him, but gave him a hut where he could serve God in solitude. After a few years he yearned for greater liberty than a hut in the shadow of a monastery could give him, and went out into the desert to live in the open air.

To restrain the natural tendency to wander, with the distractions it might bring, he marked out a few square yards and confined himself to these limits. There he began the custom, which he continued through life, of touching neither food nor drink throughout the six weeks of Lent. As always in such cases, in that of St. John the Baptist for example, and of St. Benedict, people began to come to him. They commended themselves to his prayers, they asked for advice, they begged to be instructed as disciples. Soon they so crowded on him as to interfere with his necessary hours of prayer. Then it was that the pillar idea dawned on him. He erected a platform on a pillar about nine feet in height and on this he lived, not to elevate himself, but to get out of the distractions of a loving and admiring crowd. Still they came, and in the long run his small open habitation was some fifty feet above the ground. He now added to his Lenten exercise of absolute fast the custom of standing upright for the whole six weeks. At first he had a stake fixed on his platform to which he tied himself up for fear of falling in his sleep, but having acquired the power to sleep standing he did away with this luxury.

Meanwhile the whole world was resounding with his name. For the crowds who came his platform was his pulpit, and for his disciples it was the master's chair. His voice reached millions, he converted thousands, he trained up hundreds to the higher life. He corresponded with Emperors and statesmen, and gave Emperor Leo effective advice for the Council of Chalcedon. He was ill only once in his life, and his welfare was so precious to both Church and State that the Emperor sent two Bishops to beg him to come down and be treated by doctors. He declined, and soon recovered by his own natural vitality. To apply the ultimate test, his Bishop, in the full tide of his reputation, sent an envoy to command him to leave that mode of life. The sentence had hardly passed the lips of the envoy when the foot of Simeon was on the first downward rung of the

ladder. Nor would he have gone up again if he had not been permitted.

Some might think he must have been a weakling physically. Wrong: he reached the age of seventy-two—after his boyhood eighteen years of preparation, followed by thirty-six years of achievement. Yet he was more loved than admired, and all who knew him felt that he had in him everything that was human and more that was Divine. To a critic he might, if he were not so saintly, reply: "My friend, I have done more missionary work in my life than most professedly missionary priests or bishops: if their existence is justified by that, so is mine: and what I do with my spare time is no concern of yours." The Church has always thought that his life would have been impossible without Divine inspiration and Divine aid; and for myself I will continue so to think till somebody gives me a more rational explanation. Holism should consider these extreme cases.

CHAPTER XVI

THE SUPREME WHOLE OR FORM

Those who look upon the universe from the materialistic point of view are enormously impressed by the mere hugeness of it. They may equally be impressed by its minuteness. We are so constituted that the whole universe is to us a source of indefinitely varied sense-perception in which we can never reach the limits. Nay more, owing to the gaps between our senses we know that there are mysterious possibilities close around us. If we had a sense between hearing and sight, for example, we should perceive a great deal more than we do. Would this give us new "things" or only new qualities of the things we already know? And after all, when we get beyond sensation, what is really meant by bigness and smallness? What is the value of an ordinary pebble? Practically nought. Suppose we multiply it by millions, what is its value? Still nought. If we could expand it to the size of the whole solar system, what would be its value? Still more emphatically nought. All the stars we see are merely masses of blazing rubbish. The effect of mere size is, as Coventry Patmore said, "to make dirt cheap."

There is a law in the universe, quite as fundamental as the law of gravity, and that is the Law of Waste. The pine sends out millions of pollen grains for one that is efficient, and that merely to keep up the level of the pine. The waste of attempts to reach higher levels is far greater. How many solar systems are wasted in the struggle to produce one planet with organic life? It is almost certain that such life is not possible in our solar system except on the earth. The possibilities of Mars exist only in the romances of pseudo-scientists and are the amusement of all astronomers who do not possess that American telescope. The conditions for such life are so complicated that the chances against them are almost indefinitely great. There may not be another planet in the universe that has so much as a fern or a reptile. And it does not at all follow that if there are plants and animals there are also men.

As far as we know, therefore, this earth is the living centre of the whole universe. Of old, men thought it was the physical centre as well, and one sometimes hears that the discovery of Copernicus shook the faith of Christendom. As a matter of fact, the spiritual centrality so utterly overweighs the physical that that discovery never made a jot of difference to anybody's faith.

For the Christian philosopher the fact of the Incarnation puts this view beyond question. The fact that God dwelt in visible form on this earth gives it a centrality in Creation far more assuredly than in the solar system the law of gravity gives centrality to the sun. The Law of Grace has come in to do more for the spiritual world than all the physical laws have done for the material. As He who brought it said, "I, if I be lifted up, will draw all things unto myself."

This earth is not a structural or organic whole: it is a matrix for an indefinitely varied hierarchy of wholes, the highest of which is that Organism which is gathered round the Incarnate Word. It is the last step of the progressive march of Holism from nothing to infinity. The Creative Word throughout gives to the lower the power to become something higher—matter to become life, life to become intelligence; and the final stage is concisely put by St. John, showing together the upward rise and the inevitable waste. "He came unto his own and his own received him not; but as many as received him, he *gave them power to become the sons of God.*" St. Paul describes the final unity over and over again:—"And when all things shall be subdued unto him, then the Son also himself shall be subject unto him that put all things under him, that God may be all in all" (1 Cor. xv. 28). Or again, in Eph. i. 19-23: "What is the exceeding greatness of his power toward us who believe: according to the operation of the might of his power, which he wrought in Christ, raising him up from the dead and setting him on his right hand in the heavenly places, above all principality and power and virtue and dominion and every name that is named, not only in this world but also in that which is to come. And he hath subjected all things under his feet and hath made him head of all the church which is his body and the fulness of him who is filled all in all." See also Eph. iv. 12, etc., Phil. iii. 21. and above all Col. i. 15, etc.

What apostles and theologians have taught, poets and artists have portrayed. Dante, the poet of the Christian Idea, sweeps up all Nature, all humanity, all science, all art, all philosophy, all history, and bears it with him to the Primum Mobile in order to project it all unified and sanctified into the Triune Radiance of the Godhead. Raphael in his

The Supreme Whole or Form 103

sublimest work, the "Disputa" (or Theology), reveals the same unity or wholeness; and Fra Angelico expresses, as no one else has done, both the subjective and the objective, the Kingdom within and the Kingdom without, essentially one.

Thus at the end of our review we have gone beyond General Smuts, but we are still Holistic. He may not agree with us so far, but I am sure he sees the grandeur of the idea which carries his theory to the very throne of God.

AP27'38